# The Candida diet cookbook

The candida diet food list, candida cleanse recipes and probiotic for Candida to reclaim your freedom

# Contents

**Part 1**

**Part 2**

# PART 1
# The Candida diet

## Introduction

Let me guess...you have Candida and you do not know what to do about it?

Maybe you are experiencing the itching, discharge, mental fatigue, and all the TERRIFYING symptoms of a fungal infection. And perhaps, the more you read articles and watch videos on the internet, the more confused you become. This is normal. The web is full of conflicting, unqualified advice on the VERY complex topic of Candida, thrush and fungal infections.

People claim they have the magic solution to the problem or people just try to sell you the next miracle remedy that just does not work.

The problem is that all these fake experts give you opinions and advice based on what they believe to be true without real scientific evidence.

Let me tell you something about Candida: you may have been mocked or made fun by experts when you expressed your concern about having Candida, thrush or a fungal infection. They may have said that "Candida does not exist" or that "Your symptoms are not real". Well, the truth of the matter is that Candida is ONE OF THE BETTER RESEARCHED topics in medicine. There are over 2000 scientific papers written on the topic.

It is a very REAL and very SCARY condition and with the Candida diet cookbook we are here to help you.

Let's now start to introduce ourselves:

I am Nicola Zanetti, a Registered Nutritional Therapist and Senior College Lecturer with a BSc in Biology and MSc in Human Nutrition.

I am also a 5 times Candida Amazon bestselling author and the owner of the "Nicola Zanetti Candida Recovery" YouTube channel, a platform with over 200 free to watch videos on the topic of Candida, thrush and fungal infections.

My co-author is Dominique Piperno, also a nutritional therapist, recipe master and an exceptionally talented chef.

In part 1, we are planning to give you support in all these areas:

- What is the Candida diet food list?
- What foods are allowed in a Candida diet?
- What foods are NOT allowed in a Candida diet?
- How long should you be on a Candida diet for?
- How to PRECISELY structure your day when it comes to eating to defeat Candida

In the second part of the book we will address practical, delicious recipes to support your journey against the yeast:

- Candida breakfast recipes
- Candida main courses ideas and recipes
- Candida friendly dessert recipes
- The right snacks when you have a fungal infection

This candida book here is all about supporting you, so what I will discuss will support your journey against candida in the most reliable way. As you will see in the chapters regarding the Candida diet, this kind of diet which is complex and that you need to sustain for a period of at least six months, maybe up to one year. It's important that you have all the tools that you need to sustain this commitment.

I, Nicola, will be writing the first part of the book.

In the dietary section, I will give you an introduction regarding Candida and help you to understand why Candida is such a formidable opponent and why it keeps coming back over and over and over again.

This part is crucial because you need to understand that when I give you the dietary rules, they will be extremely precise and they may seem unreasonable or strict.

The truth of the matter is that you're facing an opponent which has been around for 170 million years, so obviously something that has been around on our planet for so long is also something which is perfectly capable of surviving the harshest of challenges.

Therefore, this section will all be about what Candida does to you and what you must do to fight back, because if you stick to the rules, your situation will be much easier. However, if you start to break the rules, you are going to experience the result that everybody gets when it when it comes to Candida: they get better a little bit, and then they get worse once again. They get better and then they get worse in a never-ending cycle.

In the second section, Dominique will give you the recipes and the ideas to improve your compliance to the diet. What we're going to do with the recipes is to give you different kinds of recipes for your breakfast, for the main meals, for the snacks, for the deserts, and also some recipes for the period when you will be able to break the dietary rules as I will explain to you later in the book.

For now, just try to remember that there will be a period of time called the germination phase, where you can break the dietary rules, but you need to do it correctly.

To support you in this critical phase, we will help you also by explaining some incredibly tasty recipes made with foods that are still acceptable for a Candida diet. This section will all be about these cooking ideas; a step-by-step approach for you to be able to deal with your Candida in the best possible way.

Having read this book you will clearly understand why your plans have failed up until today, and you will be able to address those mistakes armed with new knowledge.

Grab a pen and paper and prepare to learn more about Candida. Understand that THESE FACTS are VITAL for your journey against the yeast.

Now without further ado, let's begin!

# Medical information disclaimer

## 1. Credit

1.1 This document was created using a template from SEQ Legal (https://seqlegal.com).

*You must retain the above credit. Use of this document without the credit is an infringement of copyright. However, you can purchase from us an equivalent document that does not include the credit.*

## 2. No advice

2.1 This product contains general medical information.

2.2 The medical information is not advice and should not be treated as such.

## 3. No warranties

3.1 The medical information on this is provided without any representations or warranties, express or implied.

3.2 Without limiting the scope of Section 3.1, we do not warrant or represent that the medical information on this programme:

(a) will be constantly available, or available at all; or

(b) is true, accurate, complete, current or non-misleading.

## 4. Medical assistance

4.1 You must not rely on the information on this product as an alternative to medical advice from your doctor or other professional healthcare provider.

4.2 If you have any specific questions about any medical matter, you should consult your doctor or other professional healthcare provider.

4.3 If you think you may be suffering from any medical condition, you should seek immediate medical attention.

4.4 You should never delay seeking medical advice, disregard medical advice or discontinue medical treatment because of information on this product.

## 5. Interactive features

5.1 This product includes interactive features that allow users to communicate with us.

5.2 You acknowledge that, because of the limited nature of communication through our product's interactive features, any assistance you may receive using any such features is likely to be incomplete and may even be misleading.

5.3 Any assistance you may receive using any this product's interactive features does not constitute specific advice and accordingly should not be relied upon without further independent confirmation.

# Chapter 1 introducing Candida

In this first chapter we will start by clearly introducing and defining the opponent you are facing, the yeast Candida albicans.

This part may be boring for someone who just wants to read a cookbook and learn what to do, but it is vital for me to explain to you these important aspects.

The real Candida diet is complex and has different steps and it is thus crucial that I spend some time teaching you the principles behind it.

This is to prevent you from making mistakes down the line. Trust me, I would like to just give you the recipes and the diet and be done with it.

Unfortunately, my experience with tens and tens of nutrition clients made me realise that unless a person understands fully why they are making some changes to their routine, they are unlikely to follow through with the changes after the initial period of excitement.

It is my deep desire that you will succeed in this, I know how Candida is detrimental for your body, for your confidence and for your relationships.

Please pay attention to this first part; it will be the foundation for your success.

Let's introduce your opponent now: Candida albicans is a normal, opportunistic pathogen of a human's microflora.

The oral tract, the skin, the gut and the genital area are frequently inhabited by Candida albicans.

The next issue is to understand if Candida is something common in humans and the answer is absolutely yes!

We know from scientific studies that between 65 and 80% of the human population, at least in the West where we have the majority of data from, do have Candida somewhere in their body.

When I say Candida in this instance, I mean Candida albicans.

And where in the body? As I said before, most commonly in the genital tract. Then you can experience it in the mouth and throat area, sometimes in the gastrointestinal tract and sometimes it can be on the skin and even on the scalp.

BUT Candida has the potential to grow in many other areas of the human body ESPECIALLY when immuno-challenged. This means when your immune system is not functioning correctly.

As an example, it tends to grow and lead to itchy armpits often in pregnant women.

Now, you may be wondering, okay so 65 to 80% of people in the West have Candida that seems too much. It would mean that most people you know have it right? And the answer is yes... and no.

Yes, because it is true that the majority of people you know have Candida somewhere in their body, this has been clearly proven by science.

No, because what you are calling Candida in your mind, is Candida SYMPTOMS, and clearly 65 to 80% of the population does NOT have Candida symptoms.

So what is going on here then? Where is the catch?

I will go in depth later regarding this, and why it is the case. For now, you just need to realise that Canada is present in the human body essentially in two forms. Actually there are four forms of Candida, but for now I will keep it very easy.

The first form of candida which is the one that the majority (65%-80%) of people experience, is yeast candida and yeast candida is a form of candida which is essentially harmless. In some cases it may even be beneficial, in the sense that there are some papers which seem to suggest that Candida can help the human body to absorb vitamin K.

To recap, the large majority of the population with Candida experience it in the yeast form, the yeast form is harmless.

What is NOT harmless at all, is fungal Candida!

Fungal Candida is present in about 1 to 2% of the people with yeast candida.

65 to 80% of the population in the West does experience yeast Candida, of which only 1% to 2% of those people do experience fungal Candida.

Now why is this a problem? Well, this is a big problem because fungal Candida is the type of candida that gives you the symptoms.

So, when you think about the itching, the discharge, the brain fog, the mental fatigue, the pain during intercourse, you are thinking about fungal Candida.

This is the reason why you don't hear 80% of the Western population complaining about Candida all the time.

You don't hear all of these people complaining about Candida because essentially in between these 65 to 80% only 1% to 2% actually experience those terrible symptoms.

Still, keep in mind that most people in the West do have yeast candida somewhere in their body so chances are that you may have it as well.

With this explanation let's see some biology of Candida.

# Halfway between a plant and an animal

Let's now go even deeper than before because it is of paramount importance that you realise the complexity of Candida as a microorganism.

When scientists analysed the cellular structure of Candida, they saw that Candida is halfway between animal and plant.

This is important to understand because Candida has mostly the structure of an animal cell, but it does also have some characteristics of a plant cell. The most important thing is that it has a cellular wall in the same way that a plant cell does.

It also contains something called a vacuole, which is a small organelle which is commonly present in plants and not commonly present in animals.

And now you may be thinking, wait a second I'm just buying a cookbook, what is there with these biology lessons?

Well this biology lesson is crucial for you to be able to be compliant with the diet when the situation will become difficult, and I can assure you that when you follow a diet for a period of six months up to a year, there will be difficult moments. Events such as parties, weddings, holidays etc. Times when you will be struggling with the diet and the only thing which will stop you from breaking the dietary rules and negate all of the gains  that you've made up until that point will be having a deep understanding of the biology of Candida.

This is so you can fight back. That's the reason I am introducing these two important aspects of the cellular wall and the vacuole.

As you will see in a moment, when I discuss the forms of Candida, these two tie in together and they are extremely important for the results that you want to get.

Up until now, I have mentioned two of the forms of Candida and I have explained that the yeast Candida is harmless and the fungal Candida is dangerous and gives the dreadful Candida symptoms.

The truth is that Candida can be present in your body in 4 different forms.

Let's see them:

- **Yeast form:** usually harmless and most of the time doesn't give any symptoms
- **Pseudo-hyphal form:** this is when Candida is starting to become more aggressive, the filaments are starting to grow and expand. Candida is producing many proteases to cut through your tissues. These proteases are enzymes, and essentially proteins made to cut through other proteins. Your soft tissues, such as your mouth, throat,

intestinal and vaginal tract are mostly made of proteins, and Candida can cut through them with its proteases, causing severe damage and increasing inflammation and pain.

- **Hyphal form:** the real aggressive form, the one we previously called fungal form. At this stage, Candida has grown a large net of filaments, these filaments are extending in many areas of your body and are competing with you for your nutrients, especially glucose, iron and estrogens. This is the form of Candida that gives the majority of the symptoms, so if you are experiencing them right now, let's say vaginal Candida symptoms, you have fungal/hyphal Candida.

- **Chlamydospores:** This form is hugely important and it is the reason why you may have gotten better in the past, but your Candida came back. Sometimes, when Candida is starting to expand, mainly in the pseudo-hyphal form, it does give symptoms. If a person enters into a reduced sugar diet, Candida may stop growing and hide in a spore, waiting for a moment in which food is available once again. This is done by using the thick cellular walls we introduced before. By hiding behind thick walls, Candida is essentially entering into hibernation to wait out your diet.

Let's focus more on the spores part now, as it is crucial for your success.

Now that you have seen the four forms of Candida, let me go back to the biology explanation.

The cellular walls are important because, as I said previously, Candida has the possibility of turning into spores and when it turns into spores, it is essentially becoming almost impossible to eradicate.

This is a crucial step for you, and you will see that the dietary rules in the next chapters are clearly designed to address this problem.

To make it very simple, if you go into a Candida diet, or start to take antifungals, you may be able to kill up to 80% of the fungal Candida colonies. As you do so, you will start to feel better. Unfortunately, there will be that 20% which have turned into Chlamydospores, essentially becoming unkillable.

As you start to get better, you may start to feel that you can relax the dietary rules and as you do so, the Candida spores are also starting to grow back and usually within a few months you are back to square one.

This is why you will see an important step in the dietary rules, a step which will ensure that we also destroy the Candida spores.

To close the chapter, let me address one final piece of the puzzle: up until now I have explained to you that yeast Candida is harmless and fungal Candida is dangerous. I will now explain what the reasons are that it switches from the harmless to the dangerous form.

We start from yeast Candida, this form has the shape of an egg, and it is the usual form that you see when you grow Candida in a lab under standard conditions.

When changes to its environment arise, Candida may start to move away from its original yeast form.

These environmental changes are linked to many different factors, and are the main reasons why the harmless unicellular yeast form of Candida may progress towards a more damaging form. Let's list these reasons:

- **Dysbiosis:** as we have already seen, the absence of bacterial competition makes it much easier for Candida to grow and expand into the fungal form. Additionally, as we will see in the following chapters, the different types of bacteria surrounding Candida make a massive difference in the form that Candida will take. Some bacteria keep Candida at bay, while some empower it to develop into its fungal form.

- **Elevated sugar levels in the diet:** to put this in a simpler way, the yeast form of Candida is a better form of Candida when facing a scarcity of food. Candida's main food is the sugar known as glucose, and the fungal form of Candida will thrive when in an environment rich in sugar. This is why your diet is so crucial in your journey against Candida.

- **Elevated levels of the hormones known as oestrogens:** have you ever wondered why Candida or thrush seems to be a much more common occurrence in women? This is largely because women have more elevated levels of the sexual hormones known as oestrogens. Candida uses these hormones to ease its growth into the fungal form.

- **Stress:** the more stressed you are, the more depleted your immune system will be. This is crucial as your immune system and your friendly bacteria are what keep Candida in the yeast form. Chronic stress is a big NO-NO when it comes to Candida overgrowth.

- **Vitamins and mineral deficiencies:** vitamin B3, B6, Biotin and Zinc insufficiencies or deficiencies are one of the main reasons why Candida progresses from the yeast form to the fungal form, and they need to be addressed in a real Candida programme.

So, now that you have seen the main reasons why is candy that goes into fungal Candida, you can understand why when I will give you the dietary rules. Some aspects they need to be considered in a specific way.

This closes this chapter on the biology of Candida. If you want to learn more about the yeast, I have another Candida book called "Candida Treatment for Women," and I have my YouTube channel which is called "Nicola Zanetti Candida recovery".

If you want to understand more about the science behind Candida and the reason behind certain decisions, go and check my book and my channel.

Now I will start to explain to you the principles behind the candida diet and why the diet is designed in a certain way.

After that, I will give you an exact candida diet food list, the list of all the foods that you can eat and the foods that you cannot eat.

## Dietary principles (sustainable and 'die-off')

In this part of the book, I will give you the VITAL principles behind the dietary rules and the Candida diet food list.

Right now, I need to explain to you the founding principles behind the diet.

This is because, as I have previously said, data shows that people don't really follow a diet unless they understand precisely why are they making dietary changes and the benefits of those changes.

Let's begin by introducing the first of the two key concepts behind the rules of the diet that you will see in the next chapter.

The first dietary concept is the idea of a diet being sustainable for a consistent amount of time - at least six months. Now, I know what you may be wondering: "is there a shortcut?"

This is very common. A lot of the comments that I read on my YouTube channel or my Facebook page are from people asking me about shortcuts. "Should I fast for candida?" or "Should I go in on ketogenic diet for Candida" are very common questions that are repeated in the comments many times.

This kind of mindset is quite common, and understandably so. Who wouldn't want to solve a big problem with a simple solution?

The truth is, this is a big mistake that a lot of people are making only because they're still looking for a shortcut for Candida and the shortcut for Candida does not actually exist.

In all honesty, how can you expect to find a simple solution for something that has survived in our harsh planet for 170 million years?

There is no such thing as a shortcut, or a quick solution for Candida. Once you realise and accept this, the next piece of the puzzle becomes to understand how long should you should follow the diet.

The answer to that lies in the goal that you have. Let me clarify for you: science has proven that it is basically impossible to completely remove Candida from the body of a person.

Also, completely removing yeast Candida may actually be detrimental to your health, as it seems that yeast Candida may actually support the absorption of vitamin K, a very important vitamin for your bones and the health of your blood.

So, what is the purpose of a Candida diet then? The answer is to remove and revert the fungal Candida back to the yeast Candida, to remove the chlamydospores and create balance in your body.

This balance will be achieved once your immune system and your friendly bacteria can keep Candida at bay.

The correct timing is at least 6 months, but a better choice would be one year.

This also means that if you go on a holiday, if it's Christmas time, if it's your birthday or if you're simply spending a lot of time with people who like to eat out; you will still need to follow the dietary rules.

This is crucial because the moment you don't follow the dietary rules, Candida will strike back with vengeance and you already know what that means!

You know this means that you're going to experience the symptoms once again and you don't want that. You don't want to experience the recurring symptoms one more time, right?

This is one of the most frustrating things when it comes to personal health, when you think you're getting better and then the situation gets worse once again. With Candida, I can guarantee you that your symptoms WILL come back if you don't commit for at least six months, no matter what.

The next piece of the puzzle goes like this: "is it acceptable for a person to follow a dietary regime for six months if this dieting regime is extremely restrictive?"

And the answer is obviously not. You can't fast for six months and you may struggle to stay on a ketogenic diet for six months.

The important principle here is, it will take time to improve a Candida situation so your diet MUST be sustainable.

That does NOT mean a ketogenic diet for Candida is wrong. If done correctly, it may actually work very well. Unfortunately, I have yet to see a non-athlete being able to sustain a ketogenic diet for a period of six months to one year and thus that option was discarded, favouring an easier and gentler approach.

The approach needs to be gentler for two different reasons: firstly, as I said before, to be sustainable over a period of time. This is the reason why you will see some foods, like fruits, in the diet that you may have seen as excluded in previous books or videos you watched. A limited quantity of fruit is mostly fine in a Candida diet. The yeast itself does NOT seem to be able to sustain itself with the sugar (fructose) contained in fruit and it may seem to be able to do so ONLY when paired with specific bacteria in the gut.

So you will see many kinds of fruit, in the correct quantities, are absolutely fine in your journey against Candida.

The second reason that the diet needs to gentle is incredibly important and it is due to the risks of the Candida die off.

## Candida 'die-off'

We now need to address the elephant in the room which is the candida die-off. Now this is such an important topic because the Candida die-off is the number one reason why people fail in their journey against Candida.

Let me repeat this once again: THE Number one reason! This is a pretty strong statement. Let me explain.

Let's say you're experiencing Candida symptoms: you have the itching, the discharge, the brain fog etc.

You don't feel that well, so when a human being does not feel that well, it's common practise to try and find a solution to start to get better. Obviously, you may go online and you may read about Candida solutions like anti-fungals, fasting and all kinds of quick solutions.

You then start to implement them in your routine in the hope to get better, and what often happens is within the first 10 days of your new Candida programme, you start to experience flu like symptoms: headaches; feeling tired; feeling confused; sometimes having the chills; sometimes experiencing an actual fever. So, you maybe start to wonder and think "wasn't this candida detox thing going to make me feel better? why am I feeling so bad?"

This is the CRITICAL moment! This is when people start to give up in their attempt to deal with Candida. The terrible die-off symptoms are making them feel really unwell and they may start to reintroduce more sugary foods in the hope of feeling better, and they are back with their Candida infection.

This is of paramount importance. The vast majority of the population is NOT keen to suffer in order to reach their goal. They may say they are, but when faced with a challenge like the Candida die-off, plenty of them give up.

In order for you to succeed, and this is my goal in writing this book - your total success - I need to explain to you what the Candida die-off actually is and what to do about it.

So, what's the die-off then ?

When a microorganism dies as consequence of a diet or taking antimicrobial products, this dying microorganism releases toxins into your body.

These toxins will cause all of the terrible symptoms of the die-off.

So, is the die off inevitable?

The answer is ABSOLUTELY NOT! Let me tell you why.

Consider two aspects: firstly, your body is perfectly equipped to deal with a reasonable amount of toxins. If that wasn't the case, every single person living in a polluted area like a Western city would die of cancer and this is simply NOT what actually happens.

The main organ in charge of the detoxifications of toxins, poisons and free radicals is your liver. When your liver is supported and healthy, it will protect you against the toxins that are released by the dying Candida if these toxins are in a reasonable quantity.

The key word is **reasonable**. What happens in fact when these toxins overtake the capacity of your liver of detoxifying them is known as the Candida die-off.

We can deal with the die-off if we work on the two aspects causing it:

1. The amount of toxins
2. The capacity of the liver of detoxifying them

This is why the diet and the program are designed in a specific way; its purpose is to be gentle so not too many colonies of Candida die at once and at the same time. It's designed to support the liver detoxification pathways so that your liver will protect and mitigate the die-off symptoms.

This is one of the main reasons why the diet needs to be gentle. We do not want Candida to be starting to die too quickly. If it does so, you will experience the die-off symptoms and that's undesirable.

On top of that, the diet needs to support your detoxification; your liver and the toxin elimination through urination and defecation.

This is why I will introduce some specific foods to support the liver, plenty of clear water and a good amount of fibre to really address all the challenges you may experience with a Candida overgrowth.

So, it goes without saying that not only we need to support the liver but also we need to support the elimination system which means essentially having enough water and enough fibre to actually deal with the situation.

Please pay attention to this very important step. It is not enough to just detoxify. You need to detoxify AND eliminate. Both aspects are absolutely vital when it comes to your protection against the Candida die- off.

These are the reasons why it is so important that the diet needs to be sustainable, and to address the candida die-off. It is of paramount importance not to deviate from the rules of the diet because every deviation will bring you closer to one of the issues we have just spoken about.

There is another extremely important aspect that we need to address. The Candida diet cannot be continued from day one to the end of the six months, but it needs some 'off periods' in which you break the dietary rules.

If you remember in the previous chapters, we were describing the four forms of Candida and we have also discussed the idea that Candida can turn into spores. These spores are called Chlamydospores.

These Candida spores have the possibility of essentially hiding and protecting themselves when facing a difficult situation. This means that every time Candida is in a difficult situation, every time the yeast is stressed, it can hibernate as these spores.

These difficult periods are usually when you start to take anti-microbials or when you enter into a Candida diet.

When you do so, some of the fungal colonies of Candida will die and that's when you feel you're getting better, but some of them will survive by hiding and becoming spores.

When Candida hides as these spores, it's essentially hiding behind thick cellular walls in a sort of a hibernating state, waiting for better times to come. The kind of times where you stop the diet or when you finish taking the antimicrobials. At that stage, those chlamydospores will germinate once again and when they germinate, they will slowly try to go back to the fungal form. As a consequence, they will give you the symptoms again and this is something you may have experienced in the past. It is extremely frustrating.

Is there anything you can do about it? And the answer to that question is absolutely yes, and it lies within the need to follow an 'on-off' diet.

There needs to be a moment during the diet where you starve the Candida colonies and manage to kill the majority of them, let's say 80%.

Some of them will survive by hiding as the spores, let's say 20%, and when they are in the spore form they are essentially unkillable.

The next piece of the diet needs to be a period of reintroduction of more sugary foods and this is A KEY COMPONENT of a real Candida diet.

Without this stage, you won't be able to eliminate the Chlamydospores, and Candida will COME BACK.

So, what happens when you restart eating more sugary foods?

Those spores will be tricked into germinating back into fungal Candida 'thinking' that the difficult period is behind them. This is when you strike for the second time by going back to the diet and taking your antifungals.

At this stage, following this blueprint, you will be able to really make a dent in the more resilient Candida colonies, taking you one step closer to your success.

This is where I need to remind you once again, that the diet is thoughtfully crafted to address ALL of these issues and every deviation from the original plan will reduce its efficacy.

I know that you may have already read many different versions of a Candida diet on the internet, but you need to trust the REAL science behind these rules.

I can assure you it will make a massive difference on your path to freedom.

# Candida diet rules

This programme is not a diet designed for you to lose weight. These are lifestyle changes that will need to be with you for your whole first year of your battle against Candida.

This means that in the year you dedicate to defeating Candida, you will be eating only foods listed in your programme, and you will stick to the rules 95% of the time.

Calories have not been included. You need to be responsible for what works for you in terms of calories and weight loss or weight gain.

Should you want a complete personalised step-by-step approach to deal with your Candida, you can email me at nicolazanettioffice@gmail.com.

My assistant Riccardo will answer all your questions regarding how to hire me as your private therapist.

Your programme comes down to personal responsibility. I will provide some targets to reach on a daily basis, some recommended foods, and the best way to check your progress. You must take responsibility for what you are doing, to establish whether you are reaching your targets.

## Rules:

Use Cronometer or Yazio to check the values of the food that you eat.

Should you decide to use Yazio, there is an app that makes it very easy to scan the bar codes and insert the values of the foods that you are eating daily in order to keep track of what you are consuming.

Your daily protein intake can be calculated as follows:

0.83 grams of protein x kg of body weight

For your current body weight of 55kg, the calculation is:

0.83 x 55 = 45.65

This will be rounded up to a recommended 46 grams of protein per day.

For example, a chicken breast contains approximately 30 grams of protein.

Daily **minimum** fat intake is 45 grams.

For example, 3 tablespoons of coconut oil or olive oil contains 45 grams of fat.

Daily **minimum** fibre intake is 25 grams.

For example, 8 portions of fruits/vegetables would achieve this target.

I have used kg for the programme. If you prefer stones or pounds, please use this converter to find the values that you prefer.

You shall be 100% gluten free and 99% dairy free.

You need to drink 2 litres of clean water a day. This may include glass bottled water, or filtered water. It does NOT include tap water!

To achieve this, and to have good water available on a daily basis, I would recommend **a reverse osmosis filter.** This type of filter is one of the best ways to have pure water that you can drink, use for your showers, and any other activities requiring water.

If that option is not possible, a good table filter such as a Big Berkey BK4X2 Countertop water filter system is also a very reasonable option.

If the cost of those options is prohibitive, you can purchase a Water-To-Go water bottle. It is one of the best on the market when it comes to the capacity of its filter.

**What foods to eat in the first year of a Candida diet**

This is a list of the foods that are, on average, Candida friendly.

This does not mean that they will all be suitable for you. For example, if you opt to follow a vegan diet at any time during your programme, you will need to avoid all the animal-based products mentioned here.

**Best fruits for Candida:** lemon, lime, raspberries, blackberries, cranberries, watermelons, blueberries, sour cherries, apples, especially green apples, pears, fresh apricots, pineapple, prunes, peaches, and cantaloupe melon

**NOTE:** No more than 4 portions per week (320g) and maximum 2 portions (160g) in one day.

**Best vegetables for Candida:** broccoli, kale, cauliflower, cabbage, celery, spinach, fennel, rocket and watercress, brussel sprouts, green/spring onions, red cabbage, lettuce, cucumber, artichokes, asparagus, garlic, courgettes, tomatoes

**NOTE:** you MUST reach a minimum of 5 servings/400g a day. Ideally, aim for 10 servings/800g a day.

**Best fats for Candida:** almonds, flax seeds, chia seeds, extra virgin olive oil, cold pressed flax oil, coconut oil, hemp seeds, avocado, hazelnuts and organic, grass fed ghee (ghee is the only dairy source allowed in this diet)

**NOTE:** You must consume a minimum of 45g a day of fats.

**Best complex carbs for Candida:** Buckwheat, millet, brown rice, quinoa, basmati rice, sweet potato, carrots, pumpkin, butternut squash

**NOTE:** Consume a maximum of 60g of complex carbohydrates per day, e.g. a 40g portion of rice and a 20g slice of buckwheat bread.

Other sources of carbohydrates are not included in this amount. The carbohydrates found in fruits and vegetables will not count towards these 60g of complex carbohydrates per day.

## Best proteins for Candida:

**Compulsory:** bone broth x 500ml a week, to be taken as one glass, twice a week.

Vegan option: fresh cabbage juice x 500ml a week, to be taken as one glass, twice a week.

**NOTE:** Consume 0.8g/kg of body weight per day using the following as a guide:

Wild caught oily fish e.g. S.M.A.S.H fishes (salmon, mackerel, anchovies, sardines and herrings) or trout (you MUST consume at least 250 grams of oily fish a week; OR as a vegan alternative: 25 grams a day of flaxseed or chia seeds)
Lean grass-fed organic beef, wild caught white fish (cod, sole, and halibut) egg whites, and organic lean poultry

**Best vegan proteins:** This is a tricky area as the best vegan proteins such as black beans are often associated with carbohydrates that may not be the best option for a person with Candida.

So, the best alternative here is to consider nuts and seeds as the primary source of protein, and use one serving per day of a vegan, clean protein powder to top up and reach your daily protein intake, e.g. Sunwarrior Protein Classic, or Pulsin Pea Protein Powder / Pulsin Rice Protein Powder.

## Best spices for Candida:

(one to two teaspoons per day will be sufficient)

Turmeric, ginger, garlic, oregano, fennel seeds, nutmeg, sage, thyme, rosemary

## Best fermented foods for Candida:

- (2 portions per week)
- Kimchi, sauerkraut, kefir

## Best milk substitutes for Candida:

- Calcium fortified rice milk
- Calcium fortified coconut milk
- Calcium fortified hemp milk
- Calcium fortified hazelnut milk
  Calcium fortified almond milk

So, these are the rules of the candida diet, if you have bought my previous book "Candida treatment for women," you will see that the rules are the same.

This is obviously because the science behind Candida has not changed since I published that book at the beginning of April 2020.

# The Germination phase (2 weeks)

Welcome to the Germination phase of the programme, where I will explain the rules, and the importance of the germination phase.

To explain the meaning of the germination phase, we need to recap a previous concept: Chlamydospores.

The purpose of the phase is to trick the Candida chlamydospores to resume growth, so that we can destroy them during round 2 of the programme.

You can start the Germination phase 12 weeks after you started the original diet, this germination phase will last for 2 weeks and then you will go back to the original diet for 10 more weeks.

This means that if you start your Candida diet on January the 1st, you will proceed with the diet with no interruptions until March 31st. At that stage you will do 2 weeks of Germination following the rules described here, and then you will go back to your Candida diet for 10 more weeks.

If you remember, when Candida is put into a stressful situation such as starving due to a Candida diet, it will respond by turning itself into chlamydospores. This can be thought of as a sort of hibernation, while waiting for better times to come.

The chlamydospores are very difficult to destroy, even with the best anti-Candida remedies. For this reason, we need to find a different way to deal with them for us to be able to destroy them, once and for all.

And so I present the germination phase!

This is a period of two weeks where many of the previous dietary rules will be broken to simulate the end of the sugar famine so the Candida can germinate and feast once again.

The purpose is to trick Candida into thinking that it is safe to turn back to the fungal form, but once it does so, we shall be ready to start another strong round of eradication.

It is true that Candida has 170 million years of evolution as a support, but we have science and the intelligence of the human brain on our side.

Let us now go back to our client, Juliette:

Here are the rules for the two germination phases:

In this period, you shall not take any supplements of any kind.

For these two weeks you shall resume eating a small amount of sugary foods by following the Candida diet 80% of the time and eating outside of the dietary rules 20% of the time.

For example, if you eat 3 meals per day (breakfast, lunch and dinner) you will eat 21 meals per week (3 meals per day x 7 days = 21 meals). 80% of 21 meals means 17 meals per week should be consumed following the dietary rules set out in your programme. For the remaining 4 meals per week, and only those 4 meals, you will need break the dietary rules to push the chlamydospores to germinate.

From now until the end of this two-week phase, it is acceptable to eat dairy and gluten (unless you are intolerant or allergic to one or the other) at 20% of your meals.

This means that if you are a person who has never had issues eating gluten, then in this phase you can eat some rye bread at up to 4 meals per week, should you desire to do so. If dairy gives you stomach pain and diarrhoea, stay dairy free. Do not eat something that disturbs your digestion purely because I have said that you can. Be smart!

If you do decide to drink alcohol, please limit yourself to 5 units a week.

This is a useful chart for better understanding units:

| Type of Drink | Number of Alcohol Units |
|---|---|
| Single small shot of spirits (25ml, ABV 40%) **Gin, rum, vodka, whisky, tequila, sambuca** | 1 unit |
| Alcopop (275ml, ABV 5.5%) | 1.5 units |
| Small glass of red/white/rose wine (125ml, ABV 12%) | 1.5 units |
| Bottle of lager/beer/cider (330ml, ABV 5%) | 1.7 units |
| Can of lager/beer/cider (440ml, ABV 5.5%) | 2 units |
| Pint of lower strength lager/beer/cider (ABV 3.6%) | 2 units |
| Standard glass of red/white/rose wine | 2.1 units |

| | |
|---|---|
| (175ml, ABV 12%) | |
| Pint of higher-strength lager/beer/cider<br><br>(ABV 5.2%) | 3 units |
| Large glass of red/white/rose wine<br><br>(250ml, 12% ABV) | 3 units |

**Source: NHS UK**

At the end of the 2 germination weeks, you must go back to the Candida diet 100%.

This is of paramount importance. If you start to break the dietary rules, your brain may try to sabotage you into not going back to your diet right away.

This is extremely dangerous, so as hard as it could be, after the two weeks, you go back.

This closes part one of the book. In part 2, Dominique will start to discuss the recipes and the food combinations to make your diet is extremely simple and delicious.

She will guide you with all of the ideas on how to create the ultimate Candida meal plan: what kind of foods are good; how to combine them to make dishes that are absolutely delicious, look beautiful and are, at the same time, perfect for your journey against Candida.

# PART 2
# The Candida
# recipes

# Introduction

I am Dominique Piperno, a Registered Nutritional Therapist, Specialist Chef, Cookery Tutor and Content Creator.

Food is my biggest passion and I have specialised in providing practical support to those on restrictive or therapeutic diets.

I believe cooking is a radical act of self-love, which is also a central component of your healing journey.

My aim with this book is to show you that with a little commitment and preparation, you can enjoy a feast of different foods every day, exploring a variety of textures, colours and shapes.

Your food will not only be extremely nourishing but will also make you feel like you aren't missing out on the pure joy and satisfaction that food is meant to provide.

I have incorporated the Candida Diet Food List outlined by Nicola into my recipes to make sure you have the necessary tools to fight Candida for good. Now get ready for the first set of delicious recipes ☺

# Breakfast Recipes

## Protein Smoothie

Here's an example of a nutritionally balanced smoothie with a proportionate amount of protein, fat, fibre and leafy greens. This will nourish you from the inside out, keeping you fuelled and energised for hours.

## Ingredients

(Serves 1)

350ml unsweetened coconut or almond milk

40gr frozen blueberries

50gr frozen spinach

1 scoop plant-based protein

2 tablespoons flaxseed

1 tablespoon almond butter

## How to:

Put all the ingredients in a blender and blitz until you have a smooth consistency.

Tip: When building your breakfast smoothie, start with 1.5-2 cups of green leafy vegetables of choice, such as spinach, kale, lettuce, parsley, celery or cucumber, frozen or fresh.
Make sure your smoothie is high in protein and healthy fats, and low in sugar. To achieve this, you can add nuts and seeds, but you can also utilise a

good quality unsweetened protein powder. Ideally, you are looking to achieve 15-20gr of protein for breakfast, depending on your body weight.
Add roughly 40gr of fruit, which makes ½ a portion. Keep in mind that during the Candida diet you are eating 4 portions of fruit a week - 320gr in total).

Choosing a good quality protein powder is important.
https://www.nuzest.com/products/clean-lean-protein/ and https://www.pulsin.co.uk/protein-powders/plant-based-protein.html are both great options.

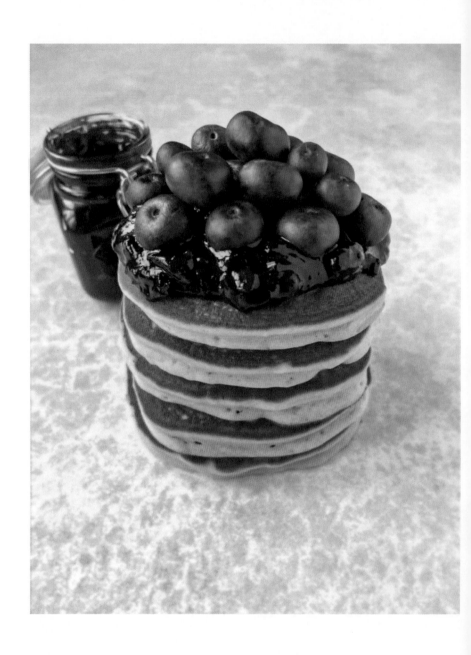

# Pancakes with Blueberry Chia Jam

These are some of the fluffiest pancakes you'll ever make! They always bring joy to the table and are the perfect weekend breakfast to savour with friends and family.
Combine them with homemade Blueberry Chia Jam and a dollop of Coconut yoghurt for pure happiness!

## Ingredients

(makes 8 pancakes-serves 2)

120gr brown rice flour

30gr potato starch

½ teaspoon xanthan gum

½ teaspoon baking powder

½ teaspoon bicarbonate soda

3 tablespoons xylitol

120ml plant-based milk of choice

2 egg whites (from two large eggs)

1 teaspoon vanilla bean

1 tablespoon extra-virgin olive oil or melted coconut oil

Pinch of sea salt

**How to**:

In a medium bowl, beat the egg whites with the xylitol for 30 seconds, then add vanilla bean, oil, and set aside.

In a separate bowl, mix rice flour, potato starch, xanthan gum, bicarbonate soda, baking powder and salt.

Combine the wet ingredients with the dry ones and pour in the milk continuing to mix until you have no lumps. For best results, let the mixture sit for 10-15 minutes.

Place a non-stick pan on medium heat and once hot, add a couple of spoons of the mixture to the pan. Cook for 2 minutes each side or until they turn golden brown.

Top with the homemade Blueberry Jam, Coconut Yoghurt (optional) and a sprinkle of flaked almonds.

**Blueberry Chia Jam**:

**Ingredients**:

250gr frozen blueberries (other berries will work too)

2 teaspoons chia seeds

2 teaspoons lemon juice

1 teaspoon xylitol (optional)

**How to**:

Simmer the frozen berries in a cooking pot, covered with a lid, until they're completely tender, for 10-12 minutes. Set aside and let cool.

Add chia seeds, lemon juice, xylitol and give it a good stir.

Serve 1 tablespoon as a topping for the pancakes.

Tip: Double the doses for the Blueberry Jam, store in a glass jar and keep in the fridge for 5-7 days. Add 1 tablespoon to your daily smoothie to increase fibre and healthy fat content, or have as a snack with plant-based yoghurt and crashed hazelnuts.

| Calories | Fat | Sat Fat | Protein | Carbs | Sugar | Fibre |
|---|---|---|---|---|---|---|
| 372kcal | 9.2g | 1.3g | 8.35g | 64g | 0.6g | 4.2g |

## Coconut Black Rice Pudding

This is the perfect comfort breakfast to feed body and soul!
The slow release carbohydrates and the fibre in the black rice will contribute to sustained energy levels and the maintenance of a healthy microbiome. Furthermore, black rice contains polyphenols which have been shown to have powerful antioxidant and anti-inflammatory properties.

### Ingredients

(serves 1-2)

100gr Thai black rice

1x 400g can of full fat coconut milk

1 teaspoon xylitol (optional)

2 tablespoons tahini paste

40gr raspberries or other fruit of choice

2 tablespoons desiccated coconut (optional)

Pinch of salt

### How to:

Soak rice in abundant water for 30 minutes and drain.

In a non-stick pan mix drained rice, coconut milk, xylitol (if using) and salt.

Bring to a boil, then reduce the heat and simmer for 25 minutes with the lid on.

Uncover and simmer for 25 more minutes at low-medium heat, until you have reached the desired creamy consistency.

Top with 1 tablespoon tahini, 20gr raspberries, 1 tablespoon desiccated coconut and serve.

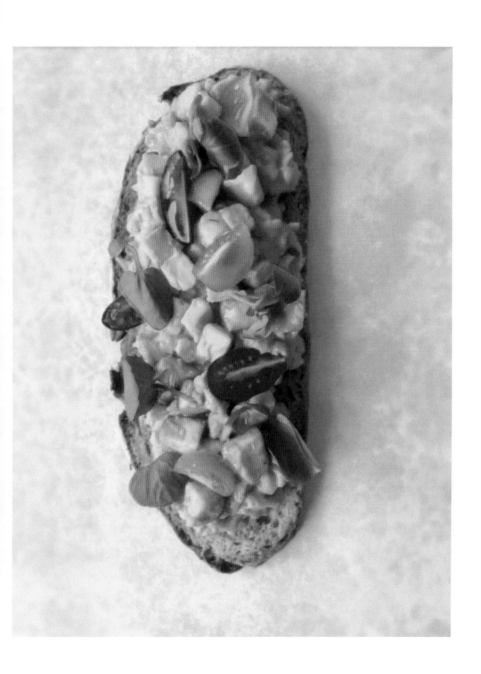

## Scrambled Egg & Avocado Toast

A classic breakfast option, quick and easy to make, yet delicious and satisfying. You can complete this dish with a portion of green leafy vegetables of choice such as broccoli, spinach or swiss chard.

## Ingredients

(serves 1)

One slice (store bought) gluten free bread

2 free range eggs (1 whole, 1 egg white only)

½ avocado

Pinch of sea salt and black pepper

A drizzle of extra virgin olive oil

A handful of cherry tomatoes

A handful of watercress

## How to:

Cut the avocado into small cubes and place in a small bowl together with the chopped tomatoes. Season with 1-2 teaspoons of extra virgin olive oil and a pinch of salt.

In a bowl, beat the eggs with a whisk and add salt and pepper.

Grease a non-stick frying pan with a little olive oil and place on low heat.

Pour in the egg mixture and let it sit, without stirring, for 10 seconds. Then stir with a wooden spoon lifting and folding the mixture from the bottom of the pan.

Repeat this procedure until the eggs are set but still slightly runny, then remove from the heat and leave the eggs in the pan for one more minute while you toast the bread.

Give a final stir and lay the scrambled eggs on the toasted slice of bread.

Add avocado, tomatoes and some watercress leaves to finish the dish.

| Calories | Fat | Sat Fat | Protein | Carbs | Sugar | Fibre |
|---|---|---|---|---|---|---|
| 325kcal | 22.1 | 3.7g | 12.8g | 21.2g | 3.7g | 6.8 |

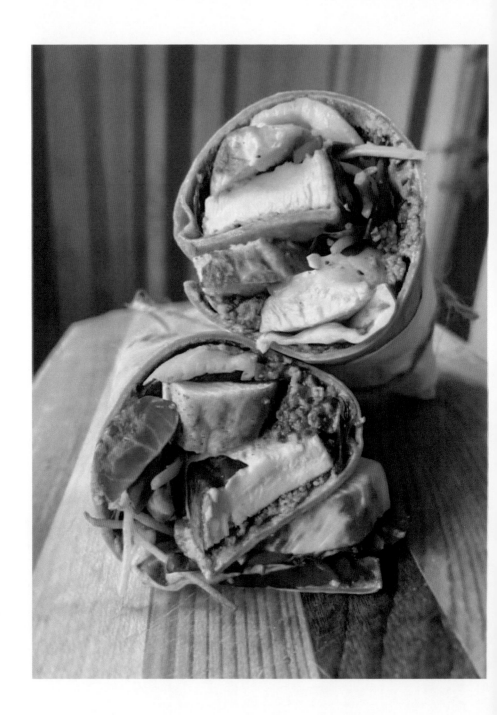

# Chicken, Pesto & Radicchio Wraps

These wraps make a delicious savoury breakfast. For extra binding, (since there is no gluten), I add psyllium, a form of fibre made from the husks of the Plantago Ovata's seeds, which helps to improve elasticity and is also known for improving blood sugar levels.

## Ingredients

(makes 4 wraps):

250ml filtered water

150gr brown rice flour

20gr psyllium husks

1 tablespoon extra-virgin olive oil

½ teaspoon sea salt

## How to:

Pre-heat your oven to 180C.

Sieve rice flour, salt and bicarbonate soda into a bowl and stir to combine, then add water and oil.

Turn into a floured surface and knead the dough for 5 minutes adding a little more flour or water if needed. Leave to stand for 15-20 minutes.

Divide into 4 portions and roll each portion into a circle, adding a little more flour to your surface each time.

Cook in the oven at 180C for 3 minutes each side.

**Fillings**

**Pesto**

(serves 4-6)

The below ingredients will make enough pesto to fill 4-6 wraps; if not using all, you can store any left-over in the fridge up to 3 days and use a topping for pasta, salads or meats.

150gr pumpkin seeds

200ml extra virgin olive oil

½ bunch fresh parsley

½ bunch fresh basil

1 garlic clove

1 teaspoon lemon juice

1 teaspoon sea salt

Pinch of black pepper


**How to**:

Add all the ingredients to a food processor and continue processing until the mixture is well blended, but still has some texture.

**Chicken breast**:

(serves 4)

4 boneless, skinless chicken breasts (approximately 120gr each)

Salt and pepper

Extra virgin olive oil for cooking

**How to**:

Place a frying pan on medium-high heat and add 1 tablespoon of extra virgin olive oil.

Season the chicken breasts with salt and pepper and cook them in the pan for roughly 4-5 minutes each side, or until golden brown.

Once ready, place the chicken on a chopping board and cut it into medium sized chunks.

**Additional**:

Complete the filling with radicchio leaves, or any other green salad of choice.

Tip: You can freeze any unused dough for later use. Get creative with the fillings, use scrambled eggs, any left-over meats, hummus and/or grilled vegetables.

| Calories | Fat | Sat Fat | Protein | Carbs | Sugar | Fibre |
|----------|-----|---------|---------|-------|-------|-------|
| 700kcal | 58.2g | 10.4g | 31g | 46g | 1.1g | 11g |

# Snack ideas

## Crispy Kale Chips:

An irresistible snack on the go, crunchy and flavourful. Be aware, if you make these, they won't last long!

## Ingredients:

(serves 6)

200gr fresh kale, stems removed

1 teaspoon melted coconut oil

2 tablespoons nutritional yeast

1/2 teaspoon sea salt flakes

1/3 teaspoon chilli flakes

## How to:

Wash the kale and dry it with a kitchen towel.

Place on a baking sheet lined with parchment paper and leave to dry completely.

Pre-heat your oven to 130C.

Drizzle the coconut oil over the kale and massage the leaves with your hand ensuring the oil is evenly distributed.

Sprinkle with the nutritional yeast, salt and chilli flakes.

Bake for 10-15 minutes depending on the strength of your oven.

Once cooked to the desired consistency, let cool and eat within a day.

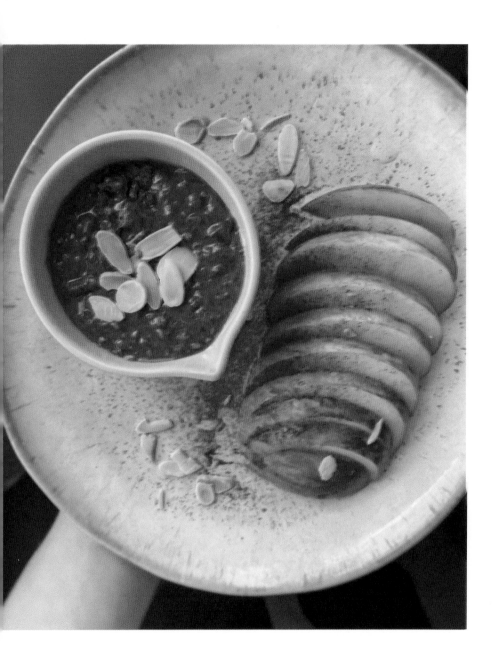

## Apple and Nut Butter:

Combine the crispy, juicy texture of the apple with the sweet, smooth touch of almond butter for a finger licking snack you will be longing for, a match made in heaven!

## Ingredients:

(serves 1)

1 organic green or red apple

1 tablespoon almond butter

A squeeze of fresh lemon juice

1/3 teaspoon cinnamon

## How to:

Wash the apple and cut it in half, then into slices.

Drizzle each slice with lemon juice and add a pinch of cinnamon.

Dip the apple slices in almond butter and enjoy!

| Calories | Fat | Sat Fat | Protein | Carbs | Sugar | Fibre |
|----------|-----|---------|---------|-------|-------|-------|
| 177kcal | 8.9g | 0.7g | 3.8 | 24.8 | 16.3g | 6g |

## Chia Pudding:

It's amazing how much nutrition and goodness one can pack into a little jar!

This chia pudding with added nuts, yoghurt (optional) and fruit, makes a wholesome snack that will help you feel the best version of yourself.

## Ingredients:

(serves 1)

120ml coconut milk

30gr crashed walnuts

2 tablespoons (30gr) chia seeds

1/3 teaspoon vanilla bean

1/3 teaspoon ground cinnamon

1/3 teaspoon ground cardamom

2 tablespoons plant-based yoghurt (optional)

1 fresh apricot, cut into small pieces

## How to:

In a little jar or a cup, mix chia seeds, milk, vanilla extract and spices altogether. Give it a good stir and make sure the seeds are completely soaked in the liquid.

Let it sit in the fridge for a minimum of 4 hours.

Once ready to serve, wash and cut the apricot in small pieces, then break the walnuts into halves.

Top the chia seeds mix with coconut yoghurt (optional), apricot pieces and walnuts.

Tip: This also serves as a handy and nourishing breakfast option. Put it together in the evening, leave it to rest in the fridge overnight and have it on the go the following morning.


## Crudités with Cauliflower Hummus

This is a simple and versatile snack you can easily carry with you anywhere.

For the crudités, you can use any vegetables that are in season, or that you favour most. Just look out for rich, vibrant colours to load up on those powerful antioxidants.

### Ingredients- Crudités
(serves 2)

Carrot sticks (made out of 1 small carrot)

Cucumber sticks (roughly 1/3 of a small cucumber)

Broccoli florets (2-3 pieces)

### How to:

Blanch the broccoli and the carrot in boiling water for 1 minute and shock in cold water to stop cooking.

Arrange in a small container along with the cucumber.

**Ingredients - Cauliflower hummus:**

(serves 5-6)

50ml water

½ large head Cauliflower

2 tablespoons tahini paste

1 garlic clove

½ teaspoon cumin powder

2 teaspoons extra-virgin olive oil

1 tablespoon lemon juice

½ teaspoon sea salt

**How to:**

Roast the cauliflower according to the instructions on page

Add it to a blender along with roasted garlic (skin off), tahini, lemon juice, cumin powder, olive oil, water and salt.

## Avocado & Walnuts

With just two ingredients, this easy combination gives you everything you want from a mid-afternoon snack: excellent fats and good quality protein.

### Ingredients:

(serves 1)

30gr walnut halves

½ small avocado

½ teaspoon lemon juice

A pinch sea salt flakes

### How to:

Roughly chop the avocado into pieces and sprinkle with the lemon juice and sea salt. Add in the walnuts.

## Desserts

Here's a light, soft cake, perfect to savour with a cup of your favourite tea. I have also made this with other berries, such as cherries and strawberries and it worked gorgeously too.

**Raspberry Cake**

**Ingredients**:

(serves 8)

170gr brown rice flour

80gr almond flour

4 large egg whites (140ml approximately)

140gr raspberries

150ml almond milk

100ml melted coconut oil

100gr xylitol

10gr baking powder (3+ ½ teaspoons)

Zest from ½ lemon

½ teaspoon vanilla bean

Pinch of salt (1/4 teaspoon)

**How to**:

Pre-heat your oven at 180C and lay a round baking tin with parchment paper.

In a large bowl mix rice flour, almond flour, baking powder and salt.

In a separate bowl, whisk the egg whites together with the xylitol with an electric mixer, add lemon zest, vanilla bean, coconut oil, almond milk and continue to mix until well combined.

Incorporate the dry ingredients into the wet ones and finally add the raspberries.

Bake for 45 minutes at 170C.

| Calories | Fat | Sat Fat | Protein | Carbs | Sugar | Fibre |
|----------|-----|---------|---------|-------|-------|-------|
| 300kcal | 18.5g | 10.8gr | 6.2g | 28.8g | 1.4g | 3.3g |

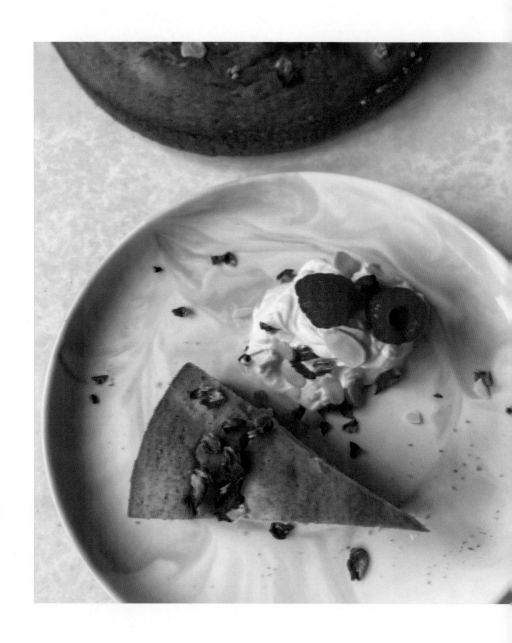

## Tahini Cookies

If you love the nutty, earthy taste of tahini you will love these cookies too.

I double the dose when I make them, as just one bunch never seems to be lasting more than a few hours!

## Ingredients:

(makes 6-8 cookies)

130g almond flour

90ml white tahini paste

1 teaspoon olive oil

1 whole egg (yolk + white)

2 tablespoons xylitol

1 teaspoon bicarbonate soda

2 tablespoons sesame seeds

## How to:

In a bowl, beat the egg and the oil together.

In a separate bowl, mix almond flour, salt, bicarbonate soda and xylitol.

Combine the dry ingredients with the egg and oil mixture, add tahini and incorporate well using your hands.

Wrap the dough in cling film and let sit in the fridge for 30 minutes.

Take the dough out of the fridge, lay a baking tin with parchment paper and pre-heat your oven at 180C.

Roll a little mixture into a ball and shape into a cookie with your hands.

Lay the cookies on the baking tin and sprinkle sesame seeds on top of each one before you bake them.

Bake for 15 minutes at 180C and let cool completely before eating.

Dip them in a Turmeric-Almond Latte for a lovely treat.

| Calories | Fat | Sat Fat | Protein | Carbs | Sugar | Fibre |
|---|---|---|---|---|---|---|
| 259kcal | 21.4g | 2.4g | 8.45g | 11.31g | 1.5g | 4.2g |

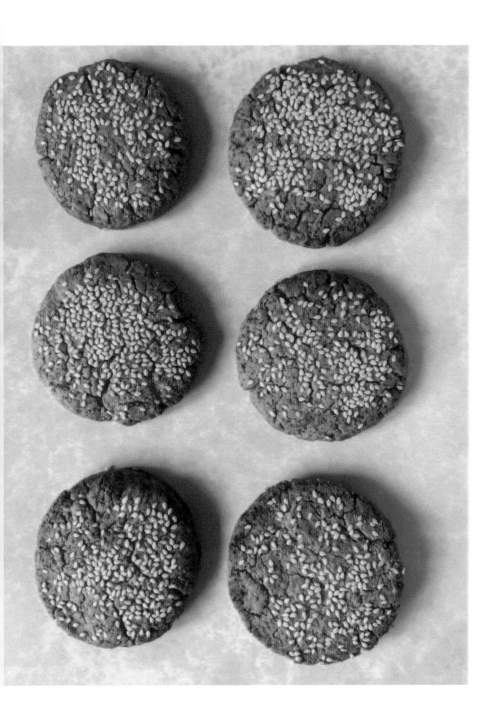

# Spiced poached pear with coconut custard

A delicate and creamy coconut custard sweetened with vanilla and topped with a deliciously spiced poached pear. Makes a lovely dessert to enjoy on a chilled winter evening.

## Ingredients - Poached pear

(serves 4)

2 pears

350ml water

2 cloves

1 fresh bay leaf

1 star anise

1 tablespoon crushed juniper berries

½ tablespoon black pepper

2 tablespoons xylitol

## How to:

Place all ingredients a part from the pears in a large heavy based sauce pan.

Stir over medium heat until the xylitol dissolves and bring to the boil.

Add the pears to the pan skin off, lay a piece of baking paper over the pears and place a small plate on top to keep them submerged in the poaching liquid.

Simmer gently for 20 minutes or until the pears are tender.

Let pears cool in the liquid and then cut each pear lengthwise so you have 4 halves.

## Ingredients - Custard

(serves 4)

400ml coconut milk (1 can)

2 teaspoons tapioca flour

2 teaspoons vanilla bean

## How to:

Add the milk to a medium sized saucepan and gently bring to just below the boiling point.

Add the tapioca flour and whisk constantly until the mix gets thick and bubbly.

Remove from the heat and whisk in the vanilla bean.

Place a strainer over a clean bowl and pour into the strainer.

Stir and push the custard through the strainer, leaving any clumps behind.

Serve warm with half a poached pear on top.

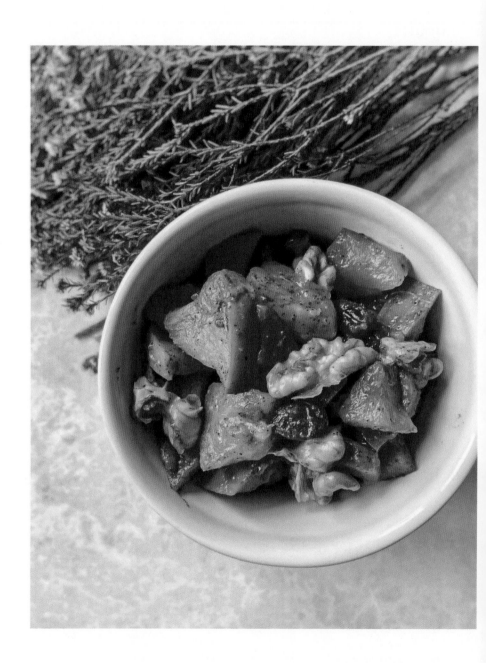

## Spiced Stewed Apples

I love to make this Dessert as soon as Autumn arrives, and the trees start to turn into endless shades of colour. It marks the beginning of a beautiful and magical season.

**Ingredients**:

(serves 4)

2 large organic red apples (skin on)

1 large organic red apple (peeled)

60ml water

1 teaspoon cinnamon

½ teaspoon ginger

½ teaspoon cardamom

30gr walnuts

20gr raisins

Pinch of sea salt

Lemon juice (approximately 1 tablespoon)

**How to**:

Peel and core the apples, then chop them into small pieces (leave the skin on, on one apple, to add more fibre and nutrients).

Put all the ingredients a part from the walnuts and the lemon juice in a heavy bottomed pan, cover and cook for 15 minutes or until nice and brown.

Take the pan off the heat and add in the roughly chopped walnuts.

Serve in a small bowl with a drizzle of lemon juice.

These are delicious both hot and cold and can be stored in the fridge up to 3 days.

| Calories | Fat | Sat Fat | Protein | Carbs | Sugar | Fibre |
|---|---|---|---|---|---|---|
| 145kcal | 5.1g | 0.5g | 1.8g | 26.6g | 19.3g | 4.5g |

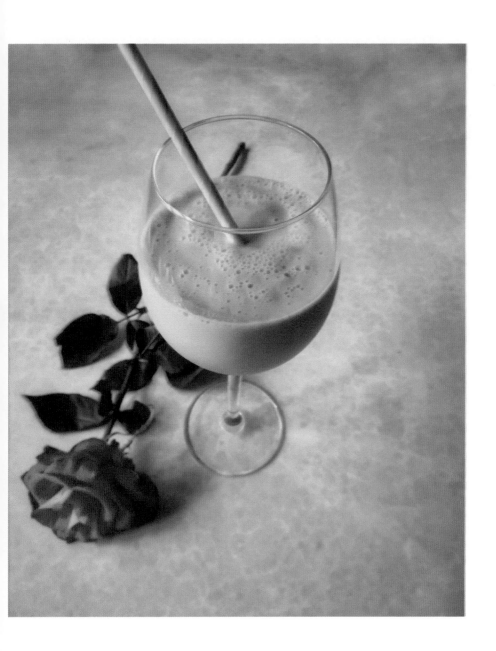

# Melon Frappe'

Melon Frappe' means summer! In fact, this is best savoured under a palm tree with stunning sea views, but of course, this deliciously creamy, naturally sweet (no)milk-shake is going to give you all the feels, even in the midst of the city chaos.

## Ingredients:

(serves 1)

180gr cantaloupe melon (frozen)

90ml rice milk

4 tablespoons unsweetened coconut yoghurt

## How to:

Take the melon, peel it, remove the seeds and cut it into pieces.

Keep it in the freezer for minimum 4 hours.

Take it out of the freezer 15 minutes before making the shake, allowing it to soften a little.

Place the melon pieces into a blender along with milk and yoghurt and blend until you reach a creamy consistency.

| Calories | Fat | Sat Fat | Protein | Carbs | Sugar | Fibre |
|----------|-----|---------|---------|-------|-------|-------|
| 142kcal | 7.3g | 5.7g | 2.3g | 20.1g | 16.4g | 2.7g |

Note: One serving of this makes just over 2 of your 4 weekly portions of fruit.

## Nourish bowls

With this section of the book, my aim isn't just to give you a bunch of recipes to blindly follow.

I would love you to learn how to combine the essential elements of a healthy plate, namely, **carbohydrates**, **protein**, **fats** and **green leafy vegetables**, so that you may continue to build balanced meals in the future, taking advantage of the endless opportunities and combinations offered by Mother Nature.

If you aim to include all the macronutrients at each meal, you will not only *never* go hungry again, but you will also achieve your health goals faster and most importantly, have some good fun along the way.

To build a nutritionally balanced plate, follow these simple tips:

1) Pick a **protein** source -aim to make this ¼ of your meal

2) Pick a **carbohydrate** source- aim to make this also ¼ of your meal

3) Now fill the remaining half of the plate with non-starchy, **green leafy vegetables**

4) Add some **healthy fat-** this should make approximately 10-15% of your meal

5) Make sure to have at least 3 different **colours** on your plate

6) Bonus add on's: Fermented vegetables, fresh herbs and spices.

I call the following meal ideas *Nourish bowls*, as they are nutritious, wholesome, colourful plates of food that will nourish you, body and soul.

I have given you ingredients and cooking instructions for each component of the plate.

Feel free to mix and match different elements of each bowl with one another, as long as the end result is a complete, satisfying meal, where all the macronutrients are present.

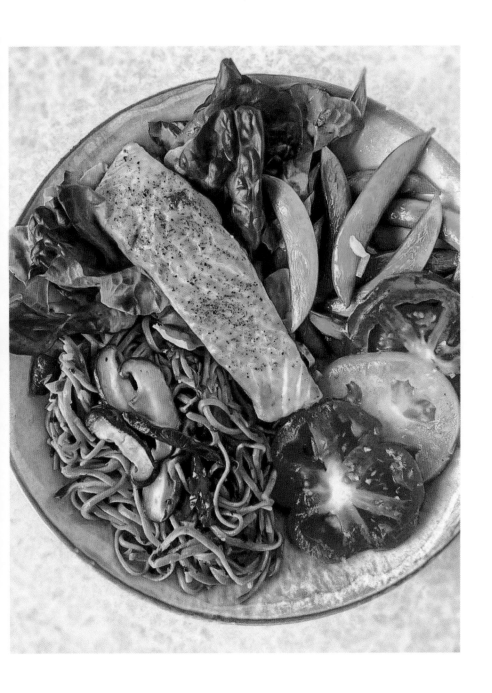

# Nourish bowl – Monday

## Carbohydrates

## Buckwheat Noodles with Shiitake Mushrooms

### Ingredients:

(serves 2)

120gr Buckwheat noodles

80gr Shiitake mushrooms

1-2 cm fresh ginger root

1 small red chilli

5 tablespoons fresh coriander leaves (approximately 15gr)

1 garlic clove

1 tablespoon olive oil

1 teaspoon toasted sesame oil for the paste + 1 teaspoon for the mushrooms

Salt and pepper to taste

### How to:

Start by making a paste for the Noodles.

Roughly chop garlic, coriander, chilli, ginger and add to a mortar and pestle together with olive oil and sesame oil. Add a pinch of salt.

For better results, add ingredients in small batches and continue to grind until they are all broken down. (If you do not have a mortar and pestle you can use a blender instead).

Roughly chop the mushrooms in small pieces.

Heat 1 teaspoon of sesame oil in a wok or large frying pan, then stir-fry the mushrooms for 4-5 minutes at medium- high heat. Add a pinch of salt and pepper.

Cook noodles as per package instructions. Once ready, transfer the noodles to the pan where you have cooked the mushrooms and add the paste from the mortar and pestle.

Stir-fry for 2 minutes on high heat.

## Protein

**Salmon fillet**

**Ingredients:**

(serves 2)

2 Salmon fillets (roughly 100gr each)

1 tablespoon olive oil

Pinch of sea salt

Pinch of black pepper

**How to:**

Season the salmon fillets with salt and pepper.

Add 1 table spoon olive oil to a large non-stick frying pan and place on medium heat.

Once the pan is hot, add the salmon fillets skin-side down and fry for 3 minutes until crisp.

Flip the fillets over, lower the heat and cook for 2 more minutes.

## Fats

### Salmon

A great source of Omega 3 fatty acids, salmon is also your main protein source.

### Extra-virgin olive oil

(used for seasoning and cooking)

## Greens and other:

### Garlic Snap Peas

### Ingredients:

200gr snap peas

2 garlic cloves

1 tablespoon olive oil

1 tablespoon freshly squeezed lemon juice

### How to:

Bring a large pot of water to a boil, throw in the snap peas and boil for 5-6 minutes.

Drain the snap peas and place them in a medium bowl.
In a small cup mix together olive oil, mash garlic, lemon juice, salt and pepper.
Pour the mix onto the snap peas and give it a stir to combine.

## Red Lettuce and Tomato salad

1 large beef tomato

120gr Red lettuce

1 teaspoon olive oil

Pinch of sea salt

## How to:

In a mixing bowl add tomato, cut into round slices or chunks and red lettuce; season with olive oil and a pinch of sea salt.

| Calories | Fat | Sat Fat | Protein | Carbs | Sugar | Fibre |
|---|---|---|---|---|---|---|
| 533kcal | 23g | 4.6g | 30.5g | 32g | 9.7g | 9g |

**Nourish bowl - Tuesday**

## Carbohydrates

**Carrot & Parsnip mash**

(serves 2)

**Ingredients**:

450gr parsnip (4 medium sized parsnips)

120gr carrots (2 medium sized carrots)

1 tablespoon olive oil

80ml plant-based milk (less if you like it thicker)

A small bunch of fresh dill

½ teaspoon sea salt

1/3 teaspoon black pepper

**How to**:

Wash and chop the parsnips and the carrots into small-medium sized pieces.

Place a large pot on high heat with abundant water and once the water boils, add the salt and pour in the parsnip and the carrots.

Cook for 10-12 minutes or until you can pierce them easily with a fork or a knife.

Drain the parsnip and the carrots and let cool slightly, before adding them to a food processor, together with oil, black pepper and an additional pinch of salt.

Process until all the ingredients are well incorporated and you have reached a smooth consistency.

Transfer the mixture back to an empty pot, add finely chopped dill, plant-based milk and let simmer on low heat for 5 minutes.

Cover with a lid and keep warm until you are ready to serve.

## Protein

### Lemon Scaloppine (Turkey)

(serves 2)

**Ingredients:**

300gr turkey breast fillets

30gr brown rice flour

The juice from 1 lemon

1 tablespoon olive oil

Pinch of sea salt

Pinch of black pepper

**How to:**

Add rice flour to a medium bowl and season with a pinch of salt and black pepper.

Add the turkey fillets and coat them thoroughly with the flour.

Heat a large frying pan on medium heat with 1 tablespoon of olive oil and once hot add in the turkey.

Cook the fillets 3-4 minutes each side, then, pour in the lemon juice keeping the heat medium-high until the meat turns golden brown and the juice has evaporated.

## Fats

**Extra-virgin olive oil**

(used for cooking and for seasoning)

## Greens and other:

**Roasted cauliflower, Mixed green salad**

(Serves 2)

**Ingredients**:

½ head Cauliflower

2 large garlic cloves

1 tablespoon extra-virgin olive oil

40gr Rocket salad/beetroot leaves/spinach

Salt and pepper

**How to:**

Pre-heat your oven at 180C

Peel the leaves off the cauliflower base and cut off the lower part of the stem.

Cut the head into four quarters and slice each quarter into 6-8 pieces.

Spread the florets out in an even layer on the baking sheet.

Add whole garlic cloves, skin on.

Drizzle evenly with olive oil and sprinkle with salt and pepper.

Place the baking sheet in the oven and let roast for 12 minutes, then turn over the florets and let roast for 12 more minutes until tender.

Wash the salad leaves and season with extra-virgin olive oil, a drizzle of freshly squeezed lemon juice and a pinch of salt.

# Nourish bowl- Wednesday

## Carbohydrates

### Roasted Butternut Squash

(Serves 2)

**Ingredients:**

180gr butternut squash

2 tablespoons olive oil or avocado oil

Salt and pepper

**How to**:

Pre-heat your oven at 180C.

Cut the butternut squash into half-moon slices, approximately 1cm thick.

Add the squash to a baking tray, drizzle with 2 table spoon olive oil, sea salt and black pepper.

Roast the squash in the oven until it's golden brown and tender for about 30 minutes, giving it a stir half way through.

## Protein

### Quinoa

**Ingredients:**

(serves 2)

40gr red or white quinoa

½ teaspoon sea salt

**How to:**

Pre-soak the quinoa in warm water for 30-60 minutes.

(Soaking is optional but it does help make nutrients more available and improves digestibility).

Drain the quinoa, add to a cooking pot and cover with salted cold water. You want the quinoa and the water in a 1/1 ratio for the best result.

Place on high heat until the water boils then lower the heat, cover with a lid and simmer for 10-12 minutes until all the water is absorbed.

Set aside and let cool for 10 minutes, then fluff it up and transfer it to a larger bowl.

## Fats

(serves 2)

### Walnuts

A great source of omega 3 fatty acids and protein, add 60gr pre-soaked walnuts to this dish.

### Extra-virgin olive oil

(used for cooking and for seasoning)

**How to:**

Pre-soak the walnuts in warm water for 30-60 minutes, then rinse and drain and lay on a kitchen towel to dry out.

## Greens and other:

### Red onion, Raw spinach

### Ingredients:

(serves 2)

125gr red onion (1 small onion)

60gr raw spinach

Pinch of sea salt and pepper

### How to:

Cut the onion into slices.

Wash and dry spinach.

Now take the large bowl where you have previously placed the quinoa, and incorporate roasted squash, spinach, red onion and walnut halves mixing well into a salad.

Garnish with ½ table spoon olive oil, additional salt and pepper, and serve.

Tip: If you don't like raw onions, you can sauté them gently in a little oil and water for 5-6 minutes, or until they're tender and juicy, before adding them to this salad.

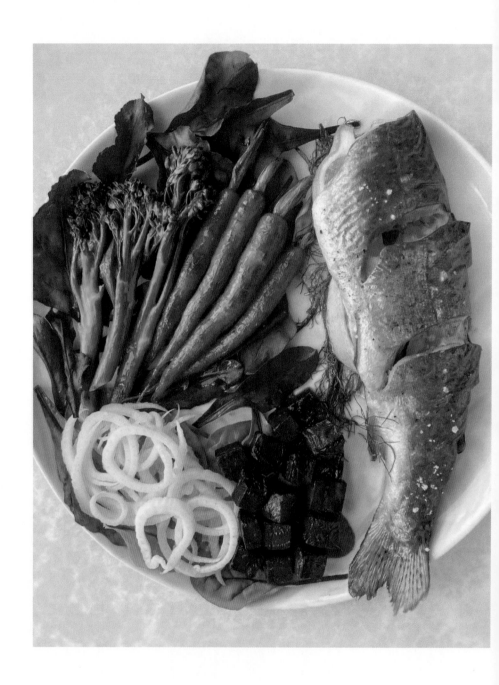

# Nourish bowl – Thursday

## Carbohydrates

### Carrots, Beetroots

### Ingredients:

240gr beetroots (2 small beetroots)

120gr carrots (2 medium sized carrots)

Seasoning: extra-virgin olive oil, salt and pepper or/and other spices such as cardamom, nutmeg, cumin and cloves.

### How to:

Once washed and chopped, both the carrots and the beetroots can be prepared 3 ways: *Steamed*, then seasoned with a drizzle of olive oil and a pinch of salt; *Sautéed* in a frying pan with a little olive oil and salt & pepper with a lid on, for 15 minutes or until they're cooked but still crunchy; alternatively, they can be cut into chunks and *roasted* in the oven for 25-30 minutes at 170C with a little olive oil, salt & pepper and fresh herbs.

## Protein

### Rainbow Trout

### Ingredients:

(serves 2)

1 whole fresh rainbow trout, gutted and cleaned

½ lemon, sliced

2 fresh dill sprigs

Coarse sea salt to taste

Pinch of black pepper

½ tablespoon extra-virgin olive oil

**How to**:

Pre-heat your oven to 200C. Lay the trout over a lightly oiled baking tray and stuff the fish cavity with slices of lemon and fresh dill.

Season with salt and pepper all over, and drizzle with olive oil.

Bake in the oven for 20 minutes until the fish is cooked through.

## Fats:

**Trout**

Rich in omega 3 fatty acids, this is also your main protein source.

**Extra virgin olive oil**

(used for cooking and seasoning)

## Greens and other

**Fennel, Broccoli**

**Ingredients:**

50gr broccoli florets

200gr fennel (1 small fennel)

Green leaves of choice: Rocket, Lettuce, Dandelion

Seasoning: Extra-virgin olive oil, salt and pepper, a drizzle of lemon juice

**How to**:

With the help of a mandolin or a knife, cut the fennel into small slices, season with olive oil and a pinch of salt.

Steam, sauté in a little olive oil, or toss broccoli in boiling water for 3 minutes, then season with lemon juice and a pinch of salt.

| Calories | Fat | Sat Fat | Protein | Carbs | Sugar | Fibre |
|---|---|---|---|---|---|---|
| 495kcal | 21g | 3.9g | 28g | 32.7g | 12.6g | 8g |

# Nourish bowl – Friday

## Carbohydrates

### Roasted Sweet potatoes & Onions

**Ingredients**:

(serves 2)

150gr sweet potato (1 medium sized potato)

120gr red onion (1 small onion)

1 tablespoon extra-virgin olive oil or avocado oil

1 fresh Rosemary sprig

Salt and black pepper to taste

**How to**:

Pre-heat your oven at 200C.

Wash the sweet potato and cut it into chunks.

You can peel it or leave the skin on, which can be easily removed once it's cooked.

Also cut the onion into 4 large pieces.

Add both sweet potato and onion to a baking tray, add olive oil, rosemary, then season with salt and pepper.

Massage with both your hands until all the ingredients are well incorporated.

Bake at 180C for 35-40 minutes giving it a stir half way through.

## Protein

## Chicken breast

## Ingredients:

(serves 2)

2 boneless chicken breasts (roughly 150gr each)

3 tablespoons extra virgin olive oil (2 tbsp for the marinade, 1 for cooking)

2 tablespoons fresh lemon juice

1 garlic clove, minced

1 fresh Rosemary sprig (can substitute 1/2 teaspoon dried herb)

1 teaspoon salt

½ teaspoon black pepper

## How to:

In a bowl, stir together olive oil, lemon juice, garlic, fresh rosemary, salt and pepper.

Place the chicken breasts in the bowl and let marinade for 1 hour (or overnight in the fridge).

Heat 1 tablespoon olive oil in a large skillet over medium-high heat.

Once hot, place the chicken breasts in the skillet and cook for 4-5 minutes on each side, until golden brown and cooked through.

**Fats**:

**Ingredients**:

1 small avocado

A sprinkle of sunflower seeds

1 teaspoon lemon juice

Pinch of sea salt

**How to**:

Cut the avocado into slices or chunks, sprinkle with 1 tablespoon sunflower seeds, drizzle with olive oil and add a pinch of salt.

**Greens & other:**

**Lettuce, Cucumber & Radish Salad**

**Ingredients**:

(serves 2)

40gr Lettuce

½ cucumber, thinly sliced

6-8 Radishes, thinly sliced

1 teaspoon olive oil

1 teaspoon lemon juice

Pinch of sea salt

**How to:**

Place all ingredients together in a large mixing bowl, drizzle with olive oil and lemon juice, sprinkle with sea salt.

| Calories | Fat | Sat Fat | Protein | Carbs | Sugar | Fibre |
|----------|-----|---------|---------|-------|-------|-------|
| 549Kcal | 24g | 4.4g | 37g | 34.3g | 15.2g | 7.4g |

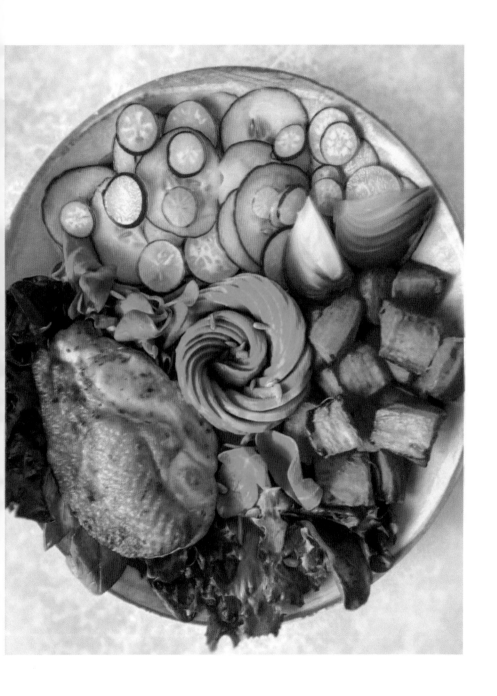

# Nourish bowl- Saturday

## Carbohydrates

## Saffron Basmati Rice

### Ingredients:

(serves 2)

120gr white basmati rice

300ml water

½ teaspoon saffron threads

1 teaspoon sea salt

### How to:

Place the rice into a sieve and rinse well in cold running water until the water runs clear.

Place water and rice in a saucepan and stir in the saffron.

Bring to a boil on medium high heat without the lid.

Once the surface is bubbly and foamy, place lid on, turn down to medium low and cook for 12 minutes or until the rice is tender and all the water is absorbed.

Remove from the stove and rest for 10 minutes.

Tip: The correct rice to water ratio for fluffy basmati rice is 1:1.5 (1 part of rice to 1,5 part of water).

## Protein

### Seabass en Papillotte

### Ingredients:

(serves 2)

2 sea bass fillets (roughly 100gr each)

½ teaspoon saffron threads

1 teaspoon fresh thyme

1 tablespoon olive oil

1 tablespoon water

2 fresh orange slices

¼ teaspoon sea salt

Pinch black pepper

### How to:

Pre-heat your oven to 180C.

In a small bowl, mix together oil with water, saffron, thyme, salt and pepper.

Lay one sheet of parchment paper on the counter and fold in half lengthwise so to make a crease.

Open the parchment paper and place one fillet just below the centrefold.

Pour the oil mix on top of the fish making sure all parts are covered.

Top the fillet with one slice of orange, cut in half.

Fold the top half of the paper over the bottom half, and begin folding tightly from the centre to the left first, and then to the right.

Repeat with each fish.

Place the packages on a baking tray and cook for 12 minutes at 180C.

## Fats:

**Extra virgin olive oil**

(used for cooking and seasoning)

## Greens and other:

**Swiss chard, Asparagus, Lambs Lettuce**

**Ingredients:**

(serves 2)

4 whole swiss chard leaves (with stems)

6 medium sized fresh Asparagus

40gr Lambs Lettuce

**How to:**

Bring a large pan of salted water to a boil.

Lower the asparagus into the boiling water and leave to cook for 2 minutes.

Add the swiss chard to the pot and blanch for 2 more minutes.

Remove chard and asparagus from the boiling water and immerse in iced water for a couple of minutes to stop the cooking process and preserve the colour.

Chop the swiss chard and the asparagus roughly, then drizzle with lemon and olive oil and add a pinch of sea salt and pepper.

| Calories | Fat | Sat Fat | Protein | Carbs | Sugar | Fibre |
|----------|-----|---------|---------|-------|-------|-------|
| 454kcal | 18.1g | 3.6g | 25.9g | 28g | 11.2g | 9.3g |

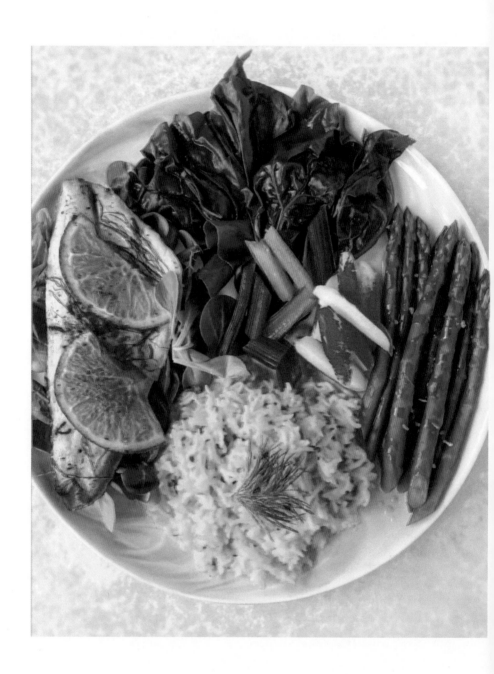

# Nourish bowl-Sunday

## Carbohydrates

### Millet

**Ingredients:**

(serves 2)

½ cup raw millet (100gr)

1 cup water

1 tablespoon olive oil

100gr cucumber

100gr cherry tomatoes

2 tablespoons chopped mint

1 teaspoon sea salt

**How to:**

Add millet to a large pan of cold salted water and give it a good stir.

Increase the heat to high and bring it to a boil.

Decrease the heat to low and cover the pot, simmer until the grains absorb most of the water, about 15 minutes.

Remove from the heat and let stand for 10 minutes.

Fluff it up with a fork, add extra-virgin olive oil, diced cucumber, tomatoes cut in small pieces, fresh mint, a pinch of black pepper, and serve.

# Protein

## Beef Sirloin steak

**Ingredients:**

(serves 2)

2 Beef sirloin steaks (roughly 220gr each)

1 tablespoon olive oil

Salt and pepper

**How to:**

Season the steaks with salt and pepper.

Oil a heavy-based frying pan and heat over a high flame.

Lay the steaks in the pan, turning every 20 seconds to 1 minute so they get a nice brown crust.

Each steak will take 4-5 min in total for medium and 7-8 min for well done.

## Fats:

## Extra-virgin olive oil

(used for cooking and seasoning)

## Greens and other:

## Rocket Salad, Grilled Courgettes, Sauerkraut

**Ingredients:**

2 tablespoons store-bought sauerkraut

1 large green or yellow courgette

40gr rocket salad

**How to:**

Place a grill pan over medium-high heat.

Wash and slice the courgette lengthwise, approximately ½ cm thick.

Drizzle with olive oil and spread it evenly on the courgettes with your fingers, then sprinkle them generously with salt and black pepper.

Grill the courgettes until tender and lightly charred all over, about 2-3 minutes each side. Make sure not to turn them too early or you will not get those great grill marks.

Drizzle the rocket salad with olive oil and add a pinch of salt.

Add sauerkraut to the plate and serve.

| Calories | Fat | Sat Fat | Protein | Carbs | Sugar | Fibre |
|---|---|---|---|---|---|---|
| 523kcal | 19g | 4.5g | 39g | 33g | 10.4g | 10.7g |

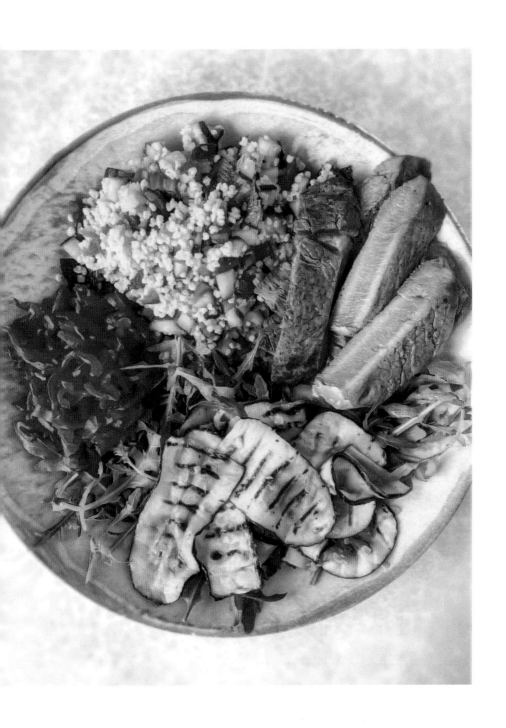

# Recipes for the germination phase

## Banana Bread

### Ingredients:

(serves 6-8)

2 medium sized ripe bananas

40ml extra virgin olive oil

1 large egg (yolk + white)

2 tablespoon brown sugar

200gr spelt four

80ml milk of choice

1 teaspoon vanilla bean

1 teaspoon baking soda

1 teaspoon bicarbonate soda

A pinch of salt

### How to:

In a mixing bowl, mash the ripe bananas with a fork until smooth and stir in oil, vanilla bean, sugar and a beaten egg.

In a separate bowl, sieve spelt flour, add baking soda, bicarbonate soda and a pinch of salt.

Combine wet and dry ingredients, add milk and mix well making sure all ingredients are incorporated.

Pour the batter into a loaf pan lined with parchment paper and bake for 50 min at 175C.

Top with apricot jam and crushed almonds (optional).

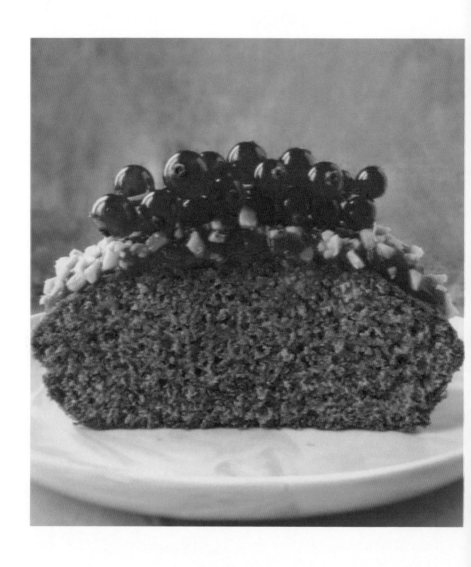

# Gnocchi with Basil Tomato sauce & Parmesan Cheese

## Ingredients- Gnocchi

(serves 4)

800g floury potatoes like Maris Piper, or King Edward

150g (store bought) gluten free flour

1 large egg (yolk + white)

## Ingredients- Basil Tomato sauce

1kg ripe tomatoes

1 teaspoon tomato puree

1 bunch fresh basil

1 shallot

2 garlic cloves

Extra virgin olive oil

Extra topping:

130gr grated parmesan cheese

## How to:

Put the potatoes in a large pan without peeling them, cover and with cold salty water and bring to the boil. Cook for 25 minutes or until soft.

In the meantime, start making the sauce by heating the olive oil over medium low heat, toss your garlic cloves until golden on all the sides and add the shallot.

Once you smell the shallot, add the tomatoes and simmer at low heat for 35-40 minutes. Add salt and pepper to taste and stir in the basil.

Pour the sauce into a blender and pulse until you've reached the desired consistency. Taste and season with more salt if desired.

Drain the potatoes, wait for them to cool down so you can handle them, remove their skin and using a potato ricer, mash the potatoes and spread them out on your work top.

Sprinkle over the flour add the egg a good pinch of salt and pepper and start mixing all the ingredients together.

Add a little extra flour if the mixture feels too sticky or if it is too dry, add an extra egg.

Cut portions of the dough then roll them like cigars and cut them into little bites.

Bring a large pan of salted water to a boil and throw in the gnocchi. As soon as they begin to float to the top, they are cooked. Strain them using a slotted spoon.

Serve them with the tomato sauce on top and a generous sprinkle of parmesan cheese.

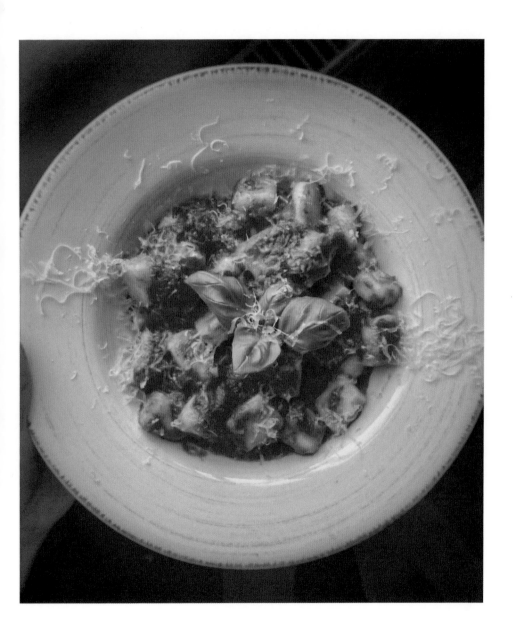

# Rice Stuffed tomatoes- Roman Style

**Ingredients:**

(serves 4)

4 large ripe but firm organic tomatoes

2 garlic cloves

8 tables spoons Arborio rice

2 medium size potatoes

2 tablespoons extra-virgin olive oil

Salt, pepper and basil to savour

**How to:**

Cut a 1/2-inch thick slice off the top of each tomato, approximately 3/4 along the circumference.

Cut and scoop the seeds, pulp, and juice from each tomato and add to a small bowl using a vegetable mill to get rid of the seeds.

Now season the mix with salt, pepper, olive oil, chopped basil and garlic.

Add the rice to the bowl, approximately 2 1/2tbsp per tomato depending on their size and let sit for 30 minutes.

In the meantime, place your emptied tomatoes in a casserole lined with parchment paper and pre-heat your oven to 180C.

Cut the potatoes into wedges and place them all around the tomatoes, season with salt, pepper and garlic cloves.

Fill each tomato with the rice & tomato juice mix previously prepared, adding any spare juice to the sides to make sure its moist.

Add basil in between the potatoes and bake for 25 min at 180C.

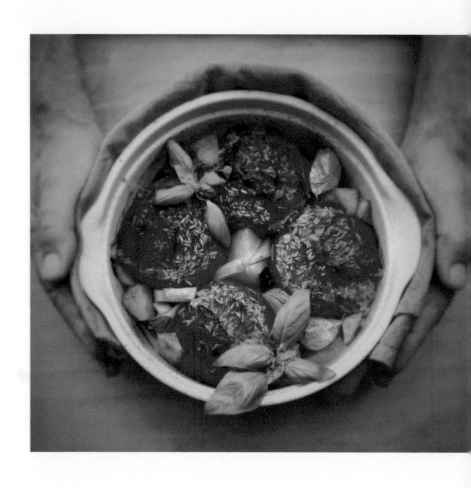

**Energy Bliss Balls**

**Ingredients:**

(serves 4-6)

130gr oats

10 dates

50gr shredded coconut

40 ml coconut oil

170ml plant-based milk

1 tablespoon raw cacao powder

½ teaspoon cardamom

Pink pitaya powder (optional)

**How to:**

Add oats, pitted dates, shredded coconut, coconut oil, milk, cacao and cinnamon to a high power blender and blend until all ingredients are incorporated.

Roll the dough into little balls with your hands, then coat them with additional shredded coconut.

Store in the fridge until you are ready to consume, or up to 3-4 days.

Tip: Roll your balls in natural pink pitaya powder, or beetroot powder to create some magic!

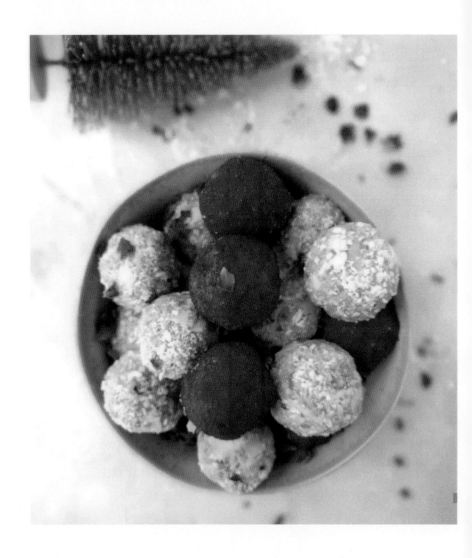

# Almond and Orange Muffins

## Ingredients:

(serves 4)

5 Eggs (egg yolk + white)

160gr unrefined sugar

2 large oranges

200gr almond flour

½ teaspoon vanilla extract

1 teaspoon baking powder

## How to:

Cut the oranges in half and boil them in a large pot for 45 minutes. Rinse, set aside and let cool.

Add them to a food processor (with the skin) and process until creamy.

In a large bowl, whisk the eggs together with sugar, add puréed oranges, almond flour, vanilla bean and baking powder. Mix thoroughly.

Bake for 25-30minutes at 170 C

## End of part 2

We are at the end of part two.

I have loved creating these recipes and I hope some of the ideas and methods outlined in this book will stay with you during and beyond your Candida healing journey.

If you would like to work with me, you can contact me on: nutrition@dominiquepiperno.com or you can find me on Instagram @Fairytale_kitchen.com.

My services include 1:1 Nutritional Therapy online consultations, bespoke meal planning, recipe creation with adjunct shopping list and private cookery tuition.

I look forward to working with you!

## Conclusion

Here you go, we are at the end of this journey. What an incredible feeling.

During the first revision, this book was supposed to be around 40 pages long, but then something happened when we were writing it... We got more and more into it and we really tried to include all the possible information you might need to manage Candida.

This book has grown with us, day after day, research after research, recipe after recipe.

With this cookbook, Domi and I tried to give you the most honest and unbiased results we were capable of.

We have spent countless hours researching and reading the best possible scientific evidence to give you the most reliable ideas when it comes to a Candida diet.

A lot of hours also were spent in the kitchen, creating recipes, and trying to find the tastiest possible foods within the parameters of the diet, and it worked!

Try the delicious recipes yourself.

To close the book, we would like to share one last word of advice. We said this before, and we will say it again: managing Candida is an ongoing process of keeping your immunity working at its best. Sometimes you might feel like easing down a bit on the protocols, and this is absolutely fine, just remember:

**NEVER LET YOUR GUARD DOWN!**

If you have enjoyed the book and feel like doing so, please go back to Amazon and leave a review for the book.

At the same time, if this book has awakened your will to know more about Candida or book me as your private therapist, you can send an email to my assistant at info@nicolazanetti.org and we can take it from there.

If you want more content on the topic of Candida, or if you just want the most delicious recipes you can follow me on my YouTube channel "Nicola Zanetti Candida Recovery" or you can follow Dominique on Instagram

**This closes the book and remember not to give up in your fight against Candida and decide today to become a relentless anti-Candida fighter!**

Yours truly

Nicola Zanetti and Dominique Piperno